This Book belongs to:

Name: ________________________________

Email: ________________________________

Phone: ________________________________

Ramped Up

www.rampedup.org.uk

www.ingramcontent.com/pod-product-compliance
Lightning Source LLC
Chambersburg PA
CBHW031325290526
45784CB00014B/1760
9781092945646